Essential Oils For Health and Healing

The Natural Holistic Remedy for a Variety of Ailments and Conditions

RON KNESS

Contents

Disclaimer

This publication is for informational purposes only and is not intended as medical advice. Medical advice should always be obtained from a qualified medical professional for any health conditions or symptoms associated with them.

Every possible effort has been made in preparing and researching this material. We make no warranties with respect to the accuracy, applicability of its contents or any omissions.

See your healthcare professional before starting any diet, health or exercise program!

Introduction

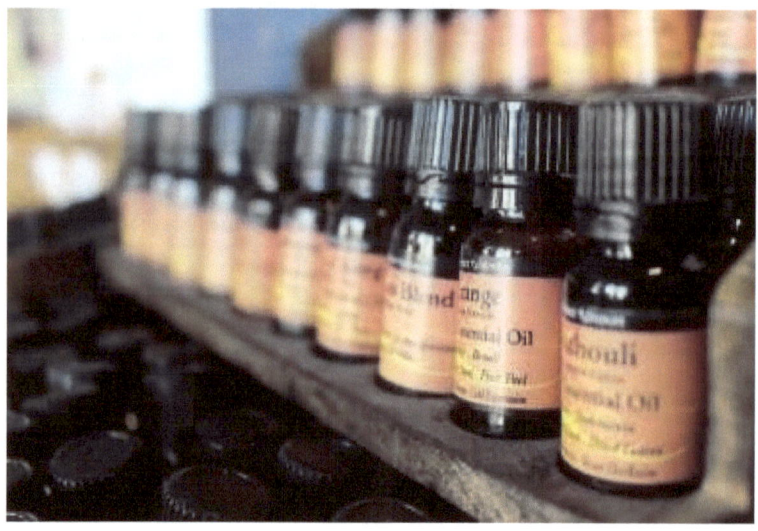

You may have heard about essential oils, especially if you look up natural remedies for physical and mental ailments, but are not sure exactly what they are. The information in this book provides a brief summary of these liquid miracle workers, how they are made, how to use and store them, and what they can do for you. Ready? Let's get started ….

What is an essential oil?

Knowing the basics of essential oils can help you understand more about how they are able to help you and encourage you to use them more often as a natural remedy. They are liquids that are extracted from parts of flowers, plants, and trees. The oils come from the flower petals, bark, leaves, seeds, roots, and fruits. Even a single drop of oil from these parts of a plant or tree can have drastic positive impacts on mental and physical ailments.

The way they are extracted is usually by steaming the plant to separate the oil from water, which is a type of distillation process. They are highly concentrated and too strong for direct contact on your skin.

Why are essential oils used?

At the heart of essential oils is their use as a natural or holistic remedy for various ailments and conditions. There is a long list of things they can help with.

While they are not meant to replace medical treatment, they can help complement and help with everything from migraines to skin conditions. Here is a short list of the many ways essential oils can help you:

- Insomnia

- Headaches and migraines

- Joint aches and pains

- Chronic pain

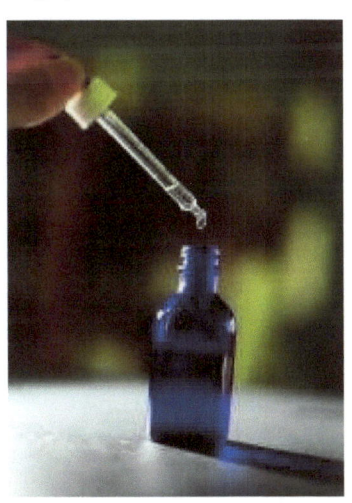

- Menstrual irregularities

- Cups, scrapes and burns

- Signs of aging and wrinkles

- Anxiety, stress, and depression

How do you use essential oils?

You have a few different options for using your essential oils. A common way is through aromatherapy, where you get the benefits from having the scent in the air, such as with a diffuser or by placing the oil itself in your bathtub, for example.

Another use is to ingest oils if they are diluted properly, which is often done when you make rose water or have it in your tea.

And then there is always using it topically on your skin when you want to get rid of acne, treat a bug or insect bite, or get a natural glow on your skin.

With essential oils, you have the option of using just one for its main benefit, such as lavender to relieve stress, chamomile for insomnia, or Frankincense for allergy symptoms. Or you can combine several different oils to make your own blends to have a different scent and help with more ailments then using one oil at a time.

Uses of Essential Oils

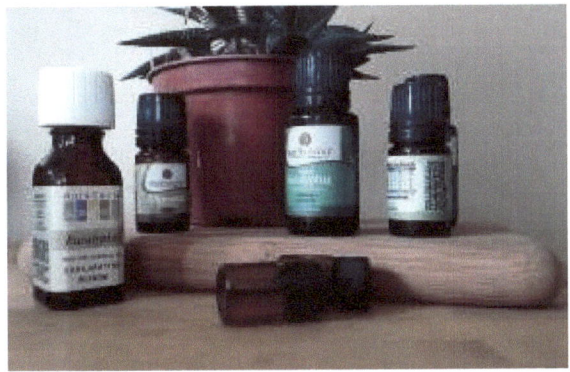

Now let's dig a little deeper into how essential oils can be used to treat various ailments and conditions.

===
For Allergies
===

If you suffer from allergies, you might be looking for a natural remedy. Essential oils are actually an exceptional way to help get rid of your allergy symptoms and start to experience relief. Here are some things to know about using them for your allergies.

How Essential Oils Can Help

Before you learn about the best essential oil blends for allergies, it helps to know exactly how the oils can help with allergies. One of the main ways they can help is by boosting your immune system.

Many of the listed oils not only boost your immune system so allergens don't affect you as much, but they can also help to fight inflammation, which is also a major contributor to allergy symptoms. Using the oils regularly will help tremendously.

Peppermint

A good essential oil to start with when you want to ease your allergy symptoms is peppermint. With peppermint, it works really great when you are already experiencing your allergy symptoms. It can help with digestive problems and the aroma is really good at helping you breathe easier, which is often a concern among allergy sufferers. Peppermint can help with skin irritation, inflammation, and most types of allergic reactions. You can either apply diluted peppermint oil around your nostrils or use it in your bath. It can also be used with aromatherapy.

Eucalyptus

Another good essential oil to try is eucalyptus, which is great for allergies and respiratory issues. Like peppermint, eucalyptus oil is also good with helping you to breathe a little better. Make sure if you are going to use eucalyptus oil for your allergies directly on your skin, you also use a carrier oil. Carrier oils are discussed later in this book.

Otherwise, it can be too strong and irritate your skin. Some good areas of your body to apply the diluted eucalyptus oil is on your neck, chest, and back. Inhaling it from a pot of boiling water is another way to get relief from your allergy symptoms.

Basil

When you suffer from allergies, it is not uncommon to have certain inflammatory responses to those allergens. This is often where many of your allergy symptoms come from. Basil essential oil can be helpful in reducing these responses so you are able to calm your body down.

In addition to this, basil essential oil helps with killing bacteria and getting rid of mold, which also helps with your different allergy symptoms. Some other ones that are good for allergies include lemon essential oil and frankincense.

===
For Anxiety
===

People who suffer from anxiety or panic attacks are often looking for ways to find relief from the attacks without turning to medications. In addition to watching your diet and getting regular exercise, it is also a good idea to give essential oils a try. Here are some of the best oils for anxiety.

Lavender

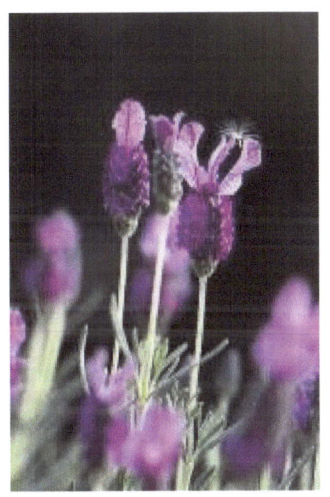

Lavender is recommended for any ailment that has to do with relaxing your body since it has such a calming effect. You can relax, get better sleep, get rid of nervousness, and even reduce your overall amount of panic attacks by using lavender. Lavender is really great in a bath when you are trying to calm down, or you can put it in an oil diffuser.

There are also DIY lotions and scrubs that can use lavender in that will also help to relax you.

Chamomile

Another relaxing and calming essential oil is chamomile. This oil helps with your anxiety, worry, and irritability. It is often recommended for people who are having trouble sleeping

7

because you will feel your body and mind start to relax when you use it. However, it is not typically recommended to people with allergy problems, so if you suffer from allergies, it is a good idea to be careful.

Rose

Rose is an essential oil you can take for stress, anxiety, and depression. It is safe whether you have allergies, are pregnant or nursing, or even if you are extra sensitive to certain oils. As with all oils, just make sure your rose oil is properly diluted or mixed with a carrier oil. You can easily add some to a pot of boiling water an inhale it to relax or add it to a footbath to start relaxing your body.

Other Essential Oils

There are a lot of other ones you can also try for your anxiety. You can use them alone with a carrier oils or create your own blends for anxiety or stress.

These oils include:

- Frankincense

- Basil

- Geranium

- Jasmine

- Clary Sage

- Mandarin

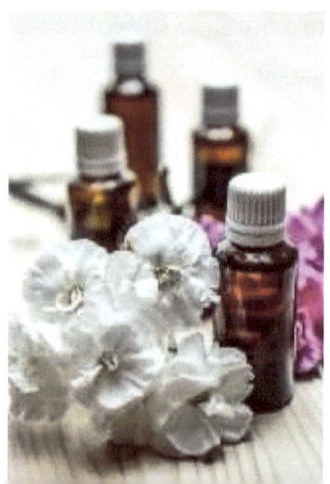

- Lemon

- Wild Orange

- Bergamot

- Marjoram

Try making your own blends with these to help with your anxiety. You can add some drops to a hot bath to relax your body and mind, use them in a footbath, or create your own body treatments.

During a panic attack, applying oils to your skin directly with a carrier oil might give you the fastest results.

===
For Arthritis
===

If you have arthritis, you know how frustrating it can be when the pain keeps you from completing normal activities. In addition to seeing your doctor for medical treatments, it is also good to try some natural remedies at home, such as with essential oils. Plants like peppermint and rosemary work very well for reducing the inflammation and swelling brought on by arthritis.

Rosemary

Rosemary oil is a soothing oil with a light floral scent that can also be used for arthritis. This is one of the top essential oils to be used for promoting better circulation. It also has anti-inflammatory benefits, so the inflammation and dwelling in your joints can be remedied with some rosemary oil. It also has anti-pain properties, which is another great reason to use it for arthritis.

For arthritis, use the rosemary oil with a carrier oil like jojoba oil, then rub it directly onto your joints.

Peppermint

Peppermint is an essential oil that works for so many ailments, but primarily body pain and inflammation issues. Peppermint oil, like rosemary oil, has anti-inflammatory properties. This means it is going to be tremendously helpful when reducing the inflammation that is leading to your joint pain. You might not be able to 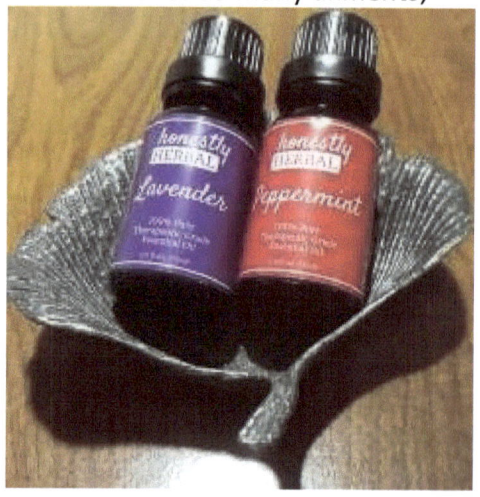 cure your arthritis, but you can bet this oil will help.

You also want to use it with a carrier oil before applying to the painful joints you have. Coconut oil is a great carrier oil to use with peppermint oil.

Turmeric

You might not hear about turmeric much, but this is an herb that is really great for arthritis. Turmeric is another anti-inflammatory herb that helps especially with rheumatoid arthritis. The herb itself is often given to people either as a supplement or to put in their food if they have arthritis. However, you can get it as an essential oil if you prefer to use it in this manner. You may also want to try a turmeric tea to help with your arthritis pain.

Frankincense

Frankincense essential oil is also good for helping with ailments that are worsened by irritation and inflammation, such as with arthritis. Frankincense oil not only reduces overall inflammation, but it can also help with the breakdown of cartilage issue, reducing the severity of it.

When you are using essential oil for arthritis, applying it directly to the skin is usually the better option. As with other oils on your skin, just make sure it includes a carrier oil. However, if adding it to a bath, it is okay to skip the carrier oil.

==
For Insect and Bug Bites
==

When you get a bug bite, it can cause stinging and burning, itching, and redness around the area where you were bit. If you use essential oils on the bite, it can help relieve many of these symptoms and speed up the healing process. Try out some of these oils for your insect or bug bites.

Lavender

You already know that lavender essential oil is ideal for anxiety, but did you know it can be really effective with bug and insect bites as well? If you have a spot on your body that is extremely itchy and starts to burn after scratching it, it is very likely a bug bite of some kind. Keep in mind not all insect bites will make themselves known right away. When you have an itch, try mixing lavender oil with a carrier oil, such as jojoba or coconut oil, then apply it to the bite. Do this for all bites and itchy spots, and you should find some relief within a few days.

Eucalyptus

Eucalyptus is an essential oil that many people are surprised by. It has benefits for your physical and mental state, helping with things like anxiety and skin conditions. It also happens to be an excellent choice when you have burns, cuts and scrapes, or various types of bug bites. It will soothe the bite so that the itching and burning isn't quite as severe, which is really all you can ask for when you have a bug bite that is bothering you.

You might also be able to apply it to your skin with a carrier oil before going outside to repel certain insects.

Tea Tree

One of the best essential oils for your skin is tea tree oil. Many people use this oil for extra moisture and to help get rid of scars. It also happens to work very well when you have a bug or insect bite.

Tea tree oil is good for boosting your immune system, which can help reduce the overall effect of being bitten by certain types of bugs. In fact, it is often given to people with bites from countries like Guatemala, China, Florida, and Australia. You want to make sure you use a carrier oil or dilute it with water, but it is good to bring with you on hiking or camping trips just in case you get a bite.

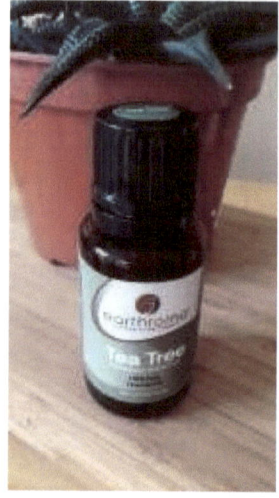

Basil and Thyme

Herbal essential oils like basil and thyme are both great for insect and bug bites. Basil essential oil is an anti-inflammatory oil, so it can help reduce the irritation and swelling around your bug bites. This further helps to help soothe the bite. You might also want to try using thyme essential oil, which reduces infection of your bug bite if the skin opens.

==
For Insomnia
==

There are few things in life more frustrating than having trouble sleeping. Sleeping is important for both your mental and physical health, and insomnia tends to get worse over time. Instead of relying on harsh medications, try some of these essential oils.

Chamomile

Chamomile tea is frequently recommended for insomnia, but not because of some magic elixir, but because of the chamomile herb. This is really effective at calming both your body and mind, relieving stress, and reducing tension.

This is why the tea is so wonderful for insomnia. The same can be said for chamomile essential oil. If you can find it, try to get the Roman chamomile oil, which has some additional soothing properties to really create a relaxing environment that is conducive to good sleep.

Ylang Ylang

If you are having trouble falling asleep or staying asleep, you might also want to try ylang ylang essential oil. This is often used to relax your mind and body, with a fruity and floral scent that is very soothing and relaxing.

When using it for insomnia, ylang ylang is best added to a blend with other relaxing scents, either to a diffuser placed in your bedroom or with a relaxing bath before you get ready for sleep.

Lavender

It should come as no surprise that lavender essential oil is helpful for insomnia. When you have trouble sleeping, it is often due to not being able to relax. This might be from certain body pains, a lot of stress and anxiety, or even depression. With lavender essential oil, it is really calming and can relax your mind and your body. As with other essential oils being used for insomnia, it is recommended in a bath, in your tea before bed, or when using a diffuser in your bedroom. Add the oil to your regular bedtime routine and you should start sleeping a little better.

Sandalwood

Sandalwood is not an essential oil often used alone, but you can easily add it to your blends when trying to improve insomnia.

This is a rich, earthy scent that is frequently used in seasonal blends because of the woodsy aroma it provides. It is a little more expensive than other essential oils, but it is great to try out when you are having trouble sleeping and other oils don't seem to be making much of an impact for you. Go ahead and give it a try and see how well it works for you.

==
For Mental Focus
==

If you have been struggling with a lack of proper mental focus and concentration, you might be looking for ways to improve it. Natural remedies are highly recommended and can be very beneficial, such as using certain types of essential oils.

Take a look at these different oils that are perfect for improving mental focus and clarity.

Rosemary

Rosemary is listed as a good essential oil for many mental and emotional conditions, from high amounts of stress, to anxiety and depression. So it should come as no surprise that it is also recommended for proper mental focus. If you have issues with your memory, concentration, or focusing for long periods of time, rosemary essential oil added to your oil diffuser is a great place to start. The scent makes you concentrate better and can help get rid of your emotional stress that might be taking away from your focus.

Basil

Believe it or not, basil essential oil is often used for mental disorders, and can work very well when you want better mental focus and concentration. It has a refreshing scent that can eliminate distraction and really help with your overall memory. Whether you need it to study, get your work done, or simply have better mental focus for various projects, basil essential oil is a really good one to start with.

Cyprus

You might not hear about Cyprus essential oil much, but you should try using it for your mental focus. This oil isn't often used for physical conditions, but it can be very effective when you are experiencing problems with your concentration or focus. If you are trying to get through college, it can help you focus when studying for exams.

If you are falling asleep at work or having trouble starting a new business, this will help with your concentration and overall memory.

Peppermint

A lot of the essential oils that work good with mental focus have earthy or minty flavors because they don't relax you like lavender and chamomile, but instead wake up your mind. You are more alert and it works similar to caffeine in the morning. There is a spicy and minty scent to peppermint that is really great when you are waking up early and don't want to keep fueling your mind and body with caffeine from coffee or soft drinks. It can also help with headaches, so that is another good bonus.

===
For Skin and Beauty
===

The oil from various plants and herbs isn't just good for your overall health, but can help with your skin and beauty as well. Take a look at some of these essential oils that will help to protect your skin from UV rays, get rid of acne and breakouts, and moisturize your skin naturally.

Ylang Ylang

When you are making your own skin or beauty products, a lot of recipes will call for Ylang Ylang. This is an essential oil that is great for reducing the signs of aging. It is often found in face and hand creams, and elixirs that are supposed to help to naturally remove fine lines and wrinkles. It is also great if you have acne or oily skin. It should be added to almond oil as a carrier if you are applying the essential oil directly to your skin.

Lemongrass

Another essential oil that is really good for your skin is lemongrass oil. All essential oils need to be diluted with a carrier oil if you are going to apply it to your skin, so try it with some jojoba, coconut, or grape seed oil. Lemongrass is best for skin conditions like acne and large pores, as well as for using as a skin toner. Most store-bought skin toner products are much too harsh for your skin, but this is light and natural, so it helps with the natural skin glow that doesn't cause irritation.

Lavender

If you have skin irritation, bug bites, or burns and scrapes, try using essential oil on your skin. Make sure you don't just use straight essential oil on your skin since it can irritate it. You should either use it with a carrier oil and apply only a small amount or make your own lavender body spray that is soothing and cooling. There are a lot of recipes for making your own spritzes and sprays that use lavender to help soothe your skin and reduce the itching and soreness of burns, cuts, and scrapes.

Geranium

An essential oil not often recommended, but highly underrated, is geranium essential oil. This is good for all skin types, is soothing, and is very moisturizing. It is good for skin that is sensitive or already irritated and won't add to the irritation. If the oil balance in your skin is keeping from a good glow and proper hydration, then geranium essential oil will be great. You can also create a face mist by adding a few drops to a spray bottle with mineral water inside.

==
For Women's Health
==

Essential oils have a lot of excellent uses, and among them, are some uses particularly for women. They can help with anything from your emotional state during pregnancy, to body changes each month during menstruation all the way through menopause.

Clary Sage

Clary sage is an essential oil that contains phytoestrogens. These are really important for all things concerning women's health, but primarily when it comes to menstruation and menopause.

Clary sage has a soothing scent that isn't overpowering, but does relax you with some aromatherapy properties. You might even find that clary sage essential oil can help to uplift your mood when dealing with irritability or depression during different parts of your menstrual cycle. However, if you have fibroids, you should reconsider using clary sage.

Lemon

Lemon essential oil has a crisp, fresh scent, that is hard not to love. Lemon essential oil still has some of the vitamin C that lemons themselves have, which provide antioxidants for your body. These can help you to feel refreshed even on a day when you have menopause or are on your period and really don't feel your best. Try adding some essential oil to a glass of warm water or tea, or making a face cream that has lemon essential oil in it.

Lavender

Lavender essential oil is often used for many different purposes, from emotional and mental health, to insomnia, and body aches and pains. It can also be great for balancing your hormones and reducing pain from menstrual cramps and other health disorders having to do with your reproductive system. If you often have headaches or stress during your period or menopause, essential oil can help you. It is also good for relieving other symptoms of PMS if you want to go the natural route.

Take a nice hot bath when you have menstrual cramps and add in some drops of lavender, or add them to a diffuser when lying down.

Peppermint

If you don't mind the minty scent of peppermint, it can be really useful for women's health. It is great when you have menstrual cramps, but mostly for your headaches or migraines. Many women experience some nasty headaches when they are on their period or going through menopause, and peppermint essential oil added to a diffuser while you lay down with all the lights off is a good way to find relief.

Using Essential Oils in Aromatherapy

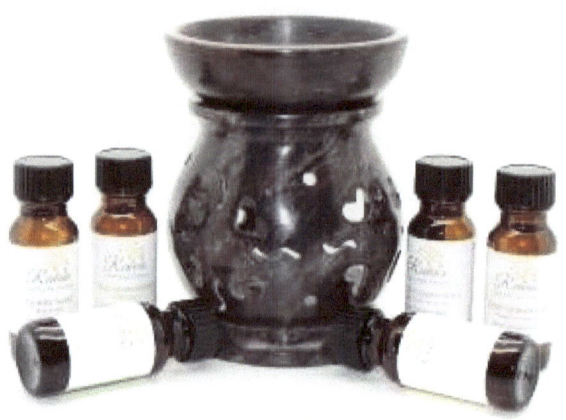

Essential oils can be used for many things, but are most often used in aromatherapy. This is when you take advantage of the scents of the oils, which can then heal your mind and body. Try some of the popular oils for aromatherapy purposes.

How Aromatherapy Can Help

Aromatherapy with essential oils helps with many different ailments, including physical and mental ones. Here are some things that you can use aromatherapy for:

- Mental health disorders like stress, anxiety, and depression

- Headaches and migraines

- Joint aches, arthritis, muscular conditions

- Inflammation and weak immune system

- To relax the nervous system

- Insomnia

- Acute or chronic pain

- Pregnancy

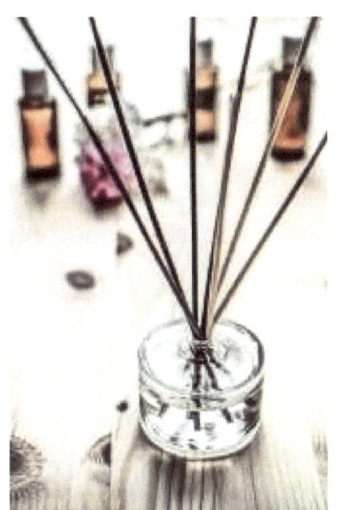

Peppermint

If you want to give aromatherapy with essential oils a try, go with something mild and minty like peppermint. This is a strong and effective essential oil that can help with anything from sore muscles to digestive issues. It is also really good for headaches and migraines, as well as congestion, cold, and flu symptoms. A good carrier oil for peppermint essential oil is grape seed oil.

Eucalyptus

Eucalyptus is also a strong essential oil that you can try using for aromatherapy purposes. With aromatherapy, you want to inhale the scented oil in order to get the full effect. Eucalyptus can be a strong, earthy scent, but don't let that fool you; this oil is very soothing and can open your airways. It is also great for relieving muscle pain, helping with asthma and congestion, and even providing dental and skin care benefits. If you prefer, you can put some drops in your bath, which still allows the benefits, without the strong scent.

Lavender

This is probably not the first time you have been told to take or use lavender products for relaxation and rest, and it won't be the last. Lavender is one of the most popular essential oils to use for aromatherapy, especially if you need help with insomnia, stress, anxiety, or depression. You will find the subtle floral scent to be very soothing and calming. Add it to your bath at night to relax enough to sleep or apply it with a carrier oil to your skin to help with burns or insect bites. It can also be used for muscle or joint pain.

Lemon and tea tree oil are other essential oils that are great for aromatherapy.

Oils That Need to be Diffused For Topical Use In Children

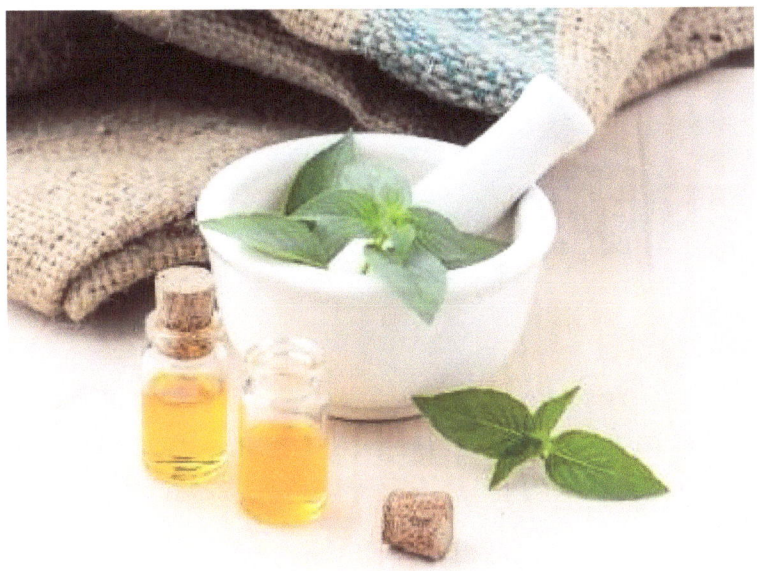

There is another category of essential oils that need to be diluted in order to use as a topical application for younger children two years of age and younger. These are safe to use as long as they are diluted with a carrier oil or with plenty of water. You should still discuss using the oils with your doctor before applying it to your baby's skin. However, some of the safer oils for topical use in younger children are:

- Bergamot

- Blue tansy

- Catnip

- Cinnamon leaf

- German chamomile

- Citronella

- Geranium

- Eucalyptus

- Lavender

- Frankincense

- Tea Tree

- Grapefruit

- Lemon

Introduce One at a Time

If you plan to start using essential oils on your kids, regardless of the method of administration, make sure you are only introducing one of them at a time. These can often be much too harsh for children, especially younger toddlers and babies. You never know what your child is going to be allergic to, so use the gentlest oils that are diluted properly, and just one of them at a time. Don't take any chances with your child's welfare, even though they are natural.

In addition to choosing the right oils and diluting or adding carrier oils, be careful how you administer the oils. On the skin can cause irritation if you don't do it correctly.

When your child is very young, you might not yet know their allergies, so introduce them slowly. Talk to your doctor if you have any concerns about using essential oils in your home or directly on your child's skin.

While usually reserved for adults, there are some instances where kids can also use them. You just need to be extra careful with the type you use and how you administer them to your children.

Essential Oils for Babies

First of all, you need to be really careful about what essential oils you use with your baby. You need to make sure they are diluted and that the proper carrier oil is used. If you fail to do this, your baby could become ill. There are also only certain ones that are good to use on babies. The oils include dill, lavender, chamomile, and blue yarrow. Make sure with chamomile, you only use German or Roman chamomile, not any other varieties.

Seasonal Oil Blends

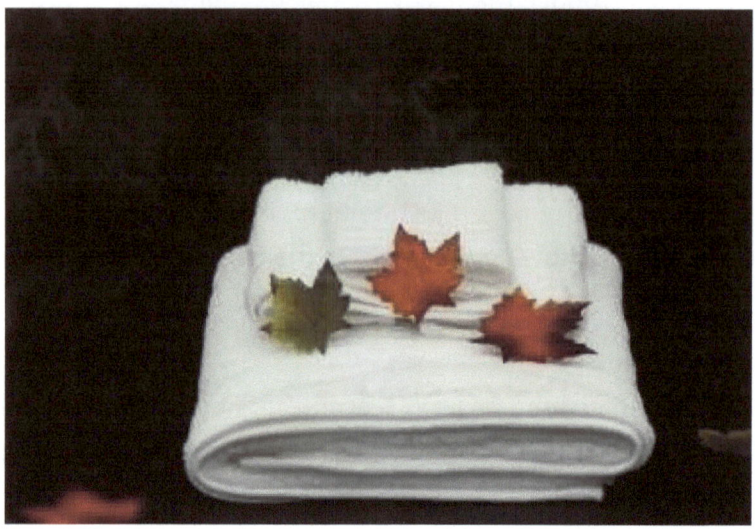

When the fall season arrives, it is a great time to get out your essential oils and put them in your diffuser. It really creates the ambiance of fall and is easy to add a wonderful aromatherapy environment to your home. Try out some of these different seasonal essential oil blends.

Candy Blend

The first essential oil blend that is good for the fall season is a candy blend. This really smells like you have just gone trick-or-treating and can smell all the different delicious and tantalizing oil scents. For a candy-inspired blend, try combining sandalwood, vanilla, and cinnamon essential oils together. You can also add in a little clove to further create a nice seasonal scent.

Ultimate Fall Blend

If all you want to smell is pure fall in your essential oil diffuser, there are some different oils that you can blend together. This doesn't include a single blend, but a list of oils you can try adding with different combinations. Remember the more drops of a certain oil, and the stronger that particular scent will be. If you want to try patchouli but not have it strong in the blend, just a few drops should be fine. Some fall-inspired essential oils to try adding include:

- Ginger

- Patchouli

- Sweet Orange

- Nutmeg

- Clove

- Cinnamon

- Lime

- Sage

- Vanilla

- Cardamom

Chai Tea Blend

If you are a fan of spicy chai tea, you will love making an essential oil blend that smells just like your favorite tea. Think about the ingredients you will normally put into your tea to spice it up, and you can probably guess what essential oils might be used for a chai essential oil blend for the fall. Some ideas are vanilla, ginger, clove, cardamom, and cassia. Make sure that even when using an oil diffuser, you combine the oils with water for your blends.

Fall Citrus Blend

In the fall, many seasonal blends will also have some citrus in them. This allows you to smell the sweet scent of your favorite citrus fruits that are in season in the fall, while also enjoying the aromatherapy in your home with a diffuser. Some oils to include in a fall seasonal citrus blend include sweet orange, lemon, cinnamon, clove, and ginger.

Add your oils to some water before putting them in the diffuser. You can also try these blends in your bath for an interesting seasonal experience.

Ways to Use Essential Oils

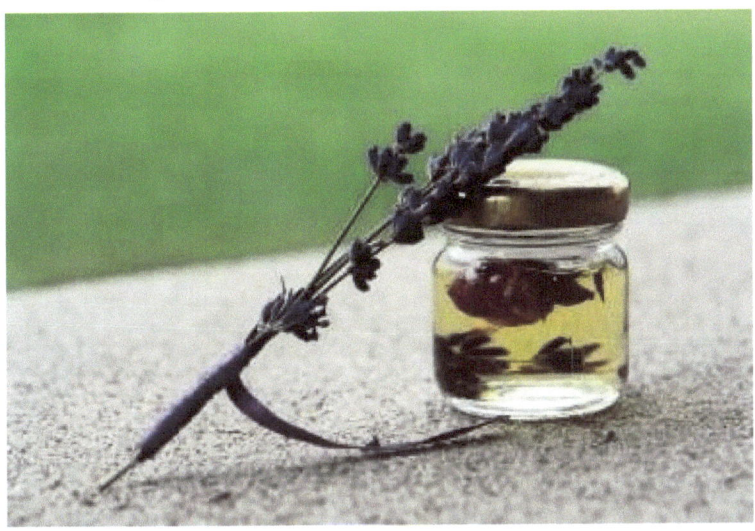

After you have learned about the essential oils you want to use for different ailments and conditions, you will then need to decide exactly how to use them. The following information provides some of the more common ways to use these oils.

Use Them in the Bath

The first way you can use essential oils is in the bathtub. This is great because you get the benefit of them both with aromatherapy by inhaling the scents, and by having them come into contact with your skin. You are able to use them without any fancy equipment, diffusers, or by using carrier oils to dilute them. With the bath, you just need a few drops of whatever oils you want to use, whether it is just one or several of them. Lavender and chamomile are great for the bath when you want to relax and de-stress, plus they help you sleep better.

Try Aromatherapy

With aromatherapy, the essential oils are inhaled and will help you heal in a variety of ways. There are blends that can work on different ailments at one time. Some things that aromatherapy helps with include inflammation, pain relief, arthritis, pregnancy pains, migraines, stress and anxiety, insomnia, and depression. A good way to use them for aromatherapy is by using a diffuser. You drop the oils into the diffuser and it puts the scent out into the room.

Apply Them to Your Skin

You can also apply the essential oils directly to your skin. When you use this method, it is often to help with a physical ailment, such as rubbing oil on your joints that are swollen and tender from arthritis, or treating a bug or insect bite. When you put them on your skin, it is very important that you mix the oil with a carrier oil.

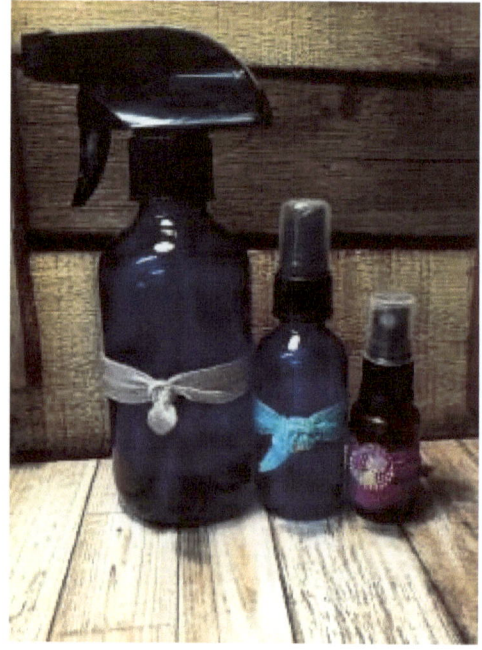

This helps to dilute the oil and prevents skin irritation from the pure essential oils. Whether treating a burn or scrape, or applying them to your skin for better moisture and glowing skin, you need to remember to dilute them.

Make Body Products

Don't forget about using essential oils for body or beauty products. The oils will further help to clear your skin, offer more hydration, or even help with healing wounds and slowing the signs of aging. Decide on what you want the body product for, then look up what each of the oils can help with. This will give you a good idea on blends to use for that skin or beauty issue.

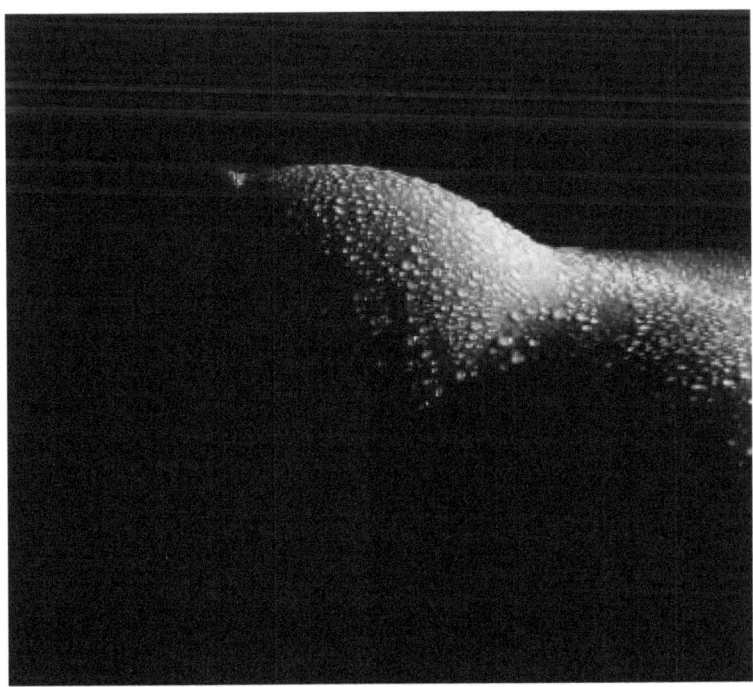

How to Use Carrier Oils

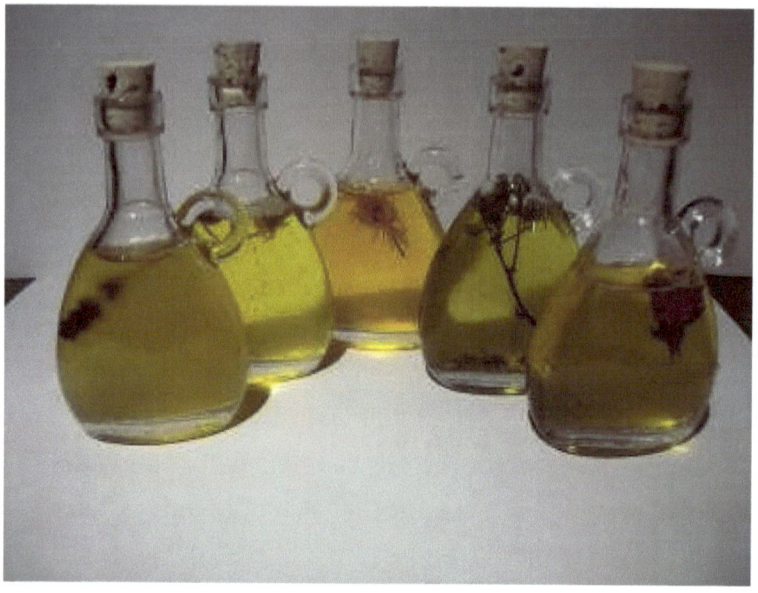

When you look up different essential oils to help with things like headaches and body pain, you probably see that if you are using the oils to be applied directly on your skin, you need to mix it with a carrier oil. But what is that exactly? Here is information on carrier oils and why they are important to add to essential oils.

What is the purpose of carrier oils?

What many people don't realize when they start using essential oils is that for the most part, oils shouldn't be applied directly to your skin. These are pure extracts from leaves and plants, which can be a little too strong for your skin. Even if you don't have sensitive skin, you could have a bad reaction to them.

Not only that, you need to neutralize the strong scent as well so they don't become overpowering. Adding carrier oils helps to dilute the essential oils to help with both of these problems. Plus, the oils provide a little lubrication and moisture for your skin, so they help in that way as well.

What are some examples of carrier oils?

Not all oils can be used as carrier oils, but many of them are great to use. Some that are commonly used include coconut oil, olive oil, grape seed oil, and hazelnut oil, hemp seed oil, and sunflower oil. Typically any oils from nuts or seeds are going to be acceptable. You should not use other forms of oil or grease in your kitchen, such as vegetable oil or vegetable shortening, butter, or margarine. You also do not want to use any type of mineral oil for application on the skin with essential oils.

Why do carrier oils help with dilution?

In many cases, oils are diluted with water, such as if you add them to a diffuser and get steam from the oil and water into the air, or you add them to your tea or a bathtub for aromatherapy. However, when they go on your skin, water doesn't work well. Essential oils evaporate into your skin very quickly, going deep into the layers of skin where it causes irritation. The same problems exists with plain water. However, oil sits on your skin for longer, so you can rub it onto the top surface of your skin with the it and it protects your delicate skin while also neutralizing the scent.

How to and Why Use a Diffuser

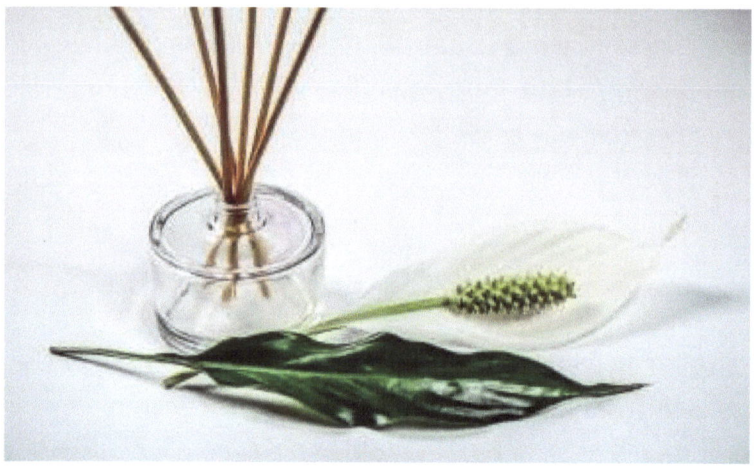

There are many different ways to use essential oils, depending on the purpose behind using them. If you are going to try aromatherapy, one excellent way to do it is by using a diffuser. Here is some helpful information on diffusers and how they are used.

Types of Essential Oil Diffusers

You should first know that there are actually a few different types of diffusers to be used with essential oils. The newer types of diffusers are cool air nebulizer diffusers, but these are definitely not the only ones available. Here is a rundown of the three most common types of essential oil diffusers:

Cool Air Nebulizer – With this type of diffuser, there is a high amount of cold air pressure that helps to vaporize the essential oils.

There is a glass bulb inside that works like a condenser, so that the oils and their benefits can be released into the air supply. This is only done in small quantities, so it provides some cool air and the scent of the oils, but it doesn't damage anyone's lungs. While cool air nebulizers are quality diffusers that work well for a wide range of benefits, they can't handle the stronger essential oils like sandalwood.

Electric Heat – You might also find an electric diffuser that is a little smaller and has a slightly simpler system than the nebulizer diffuser. With the electric heat diffusers, they have a chamber with absorbent pads on the inside. The oils are placed on the pads and heat after plugging it in will help the oils get into the air. These are really easy to use and do work good on the stronger oils, like ylang ylang and sandalwood.

Candle – There are also candle diffusers, which look similar to a tart warmer. There is a glass container that holds a small candle on the bottom and you place the oils on the tray on the top. The heat works similar to the electric heat diffuser to release the scent of the oils.

Tips For Using the Diffuser

Make sure you read the instructions manual for the type of diffuser you are using. These instructions are going to be for a nebulizer essential oil s diffuser. For this type of diffuser, you will first need to assemble it, then plug it in. You will need to put about 15-20 total drops into the chamber, but this is total for all oils. If you are using more than one type of oil, only put about 5 drops of each one.

Tips for Storing Essential Oils

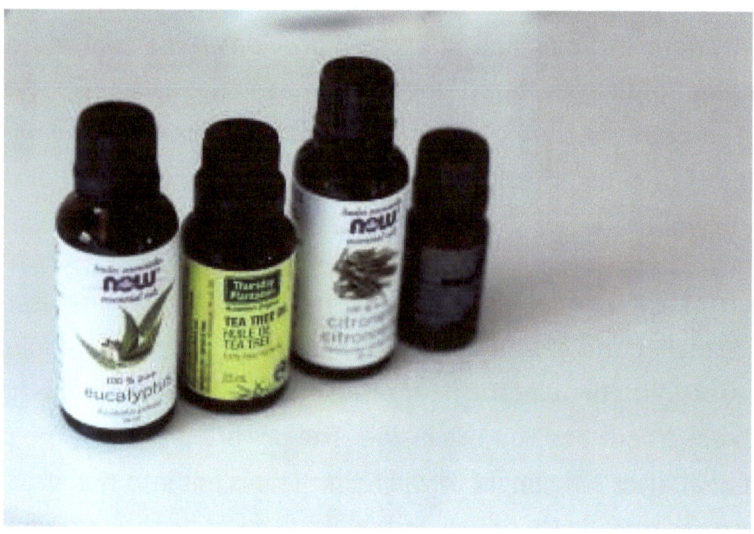

When you start collecting essential oils for beauty, skin care, or natural health, you will need to find a good place to put them. When you have just one or two, it is easy to put them on the counter or in a medicine cabinet, but you should know the proper way to store them so that they can last as long as possible.

Keep the Oils in Their Original Bottles

The bottles that your oils come in are not just there for decoration or convenience; these bottles are made specifically for holding essential oils. These oils need to be placed in dark glass bottles, since it helps reduce UV light that can cause damage to the liquid. You will most likely get your oils in these dark bottles, so try to keep them in there. If you are making blends, pour the finished blend into another dark-colored glass bottle.

You can usually get them at just about any store that sells essential oils or DIY products, from crafts stores to big box stores. Also try health food stores or look online.

Place the Bottles in a Cool, Dry Place

Once you have them in the right bottle, ensure they are never left out in the sun. If your kitchen or bathroom has a window and the sun can get in, you need to put the bottles inside a cupboard where it is dark, cool, and dry. Don't put them near the edge of the shelves in whatever cupboard you store them so you don't accidentally knock them down when opening up the cupboard or medicine cabinet door. They can be a danger for children to ingest, so try to choose a cabinet up high or one that is locked where nobody can get to them.

Store Your Carrier Oils in the Fridge

For your carrier oils, they are similar to other oil that you have for cooking. They need to be kept in room temperature, preferably in a cabinet and not left out on the counter. This is going to help prevent them from spoiling. However, if it gets hot inside your home, the pantry or cupboard is not enough to protect them. In this case, it is better to start them in the refrigerator. If you open a carrier oil bottle and it smells sour, then it has gone bad and needs to be replaced.

Final Thoughts

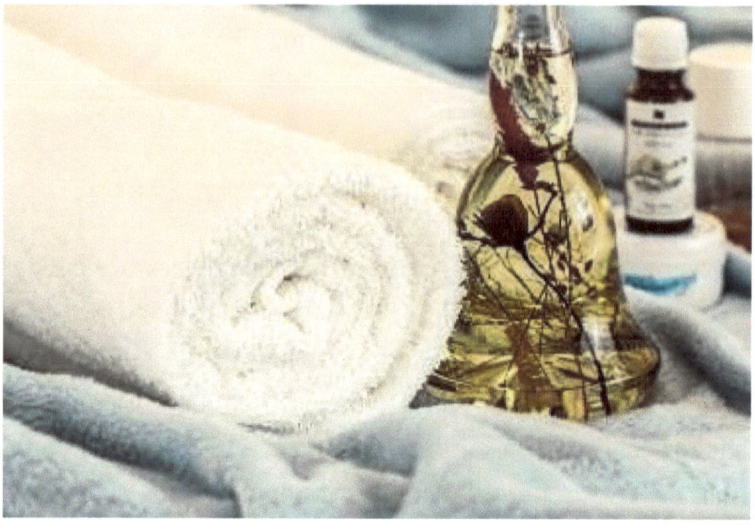

In a previous chapter, we covered which oils to use for various ailments and conditions. As a final chapter, I wanted to list the oil and then its uses as a cross reference. As noted in the essential oils chapter, there are some oils and things you should include in a basic care kit to get you started. Here are some of the basic oils and their uses to get you started:

Lavender

There are many uses for essential lavender oil. These are just some of them. You can likely find even more uses for lavender oil if you wanted to.

Calming – Inhale a few drops of lavender oil to help create calmness. You can use it in crowded places, in your car, or office discretely. Just put a few drops on a cotton ball and smell it, or put in a diffuser to spritz the air.

You can also put it into lotion to rub on your hands and arms, inhaling as you do to enhance calmness. It will also help you get to sleep at night.

Insect Bites, Minor Cuts & Burns, Skin Issues, Cold Sores & Dandruff -- Putting a couple drops of lavender oil into carrier oil then rubbing it into your skin, scalp or on a bit on irritation can help calm the skin and heal the problem.

Nausea & Motion Sickness -- Put a couple drops of lavender oil behind your ears to help with motion sickness and nausea.

Nosebleeds – Make a compress with a drop or two of lavender oil on a tissue or cloth and then press it under the base of the nose to help stop the bleeding.

In Food – While you should be careful about eating essential oils because you need to be sure to buy the right kind, lavender oil is especially good in recipes and iced tea. It can help reduce allergies and more.

Lavender is an amazing essential oil with many uses. Most people also love the smell so you can safely use it to help an entire household relax. On a side note lavender is exceptionally easy to grow requiring virtually no watering or care after you plant it.

Tea Tree

You can use tea tree oil to treat everything from acne to sunburn if you know how.

Acne – Treat your acne with a couple drops added to lotion and then apply to the blemishes every night to help treat them.

Athlete's Foot – Add some to warm water to soak your feet in. This will help cure your athlete's foot as well as help treat other types of yeast infection related illnesses.

Antiseptic – Great for use on cuts, burns and other skin problems because it kills germs and prevents infection.

Chest Congestion – Put some tea tree oil into a vaporizer to help loosen chest congestion.

Using tea tree oil in these treatments will work wonders. Some people even say tea tree oil can treat headaches, colds and even lice.

Peppermint

There are so many uses for peppermint oil when it comes to aromatherapy. One of the most used essential oils; it can treat everything from a cold to sore muscles.

Energy – When you are feeling tired during the day, just take a whiff of peppermint oil and it will pick you up fast. No need for caffeine.

Great for road trips, studying, school and more – try adding a few drops to your shampoo for a morning pick me up that won't quit.

Diet Aid – If you are hungry inhaling peppermint oil can help reduce cravings and hunger. Just put a drop or two on your temples or collarbone whenever you feel hungry to help get yourself back under control.

Muscle Care – Put a few drops of peppermint in carrier oils like sweet almond oil and rub directly on the sore muscles for best results to reduce pain and improve healing.

Focus & Concentration – Some people claim that smelling peppermint oil can help people and children with ADHD gain focus and concentrate better on tasks.

There are many more ways to use peppermint oil such as to help with teething, colic, balancing hormones and more. As you learn more about the uses of peppermint oil you'll definitely want to keep it around.

Chamomile

Universally thought of safe by doctors and practitioners alike, chamomile is used for an anti-inflammatory calming action.

Calming – Put a few drops in some hot water, place a towel over your head and the bowl to inhale the steam.

Bruises, bites, stings, skin irritation – Make a compress by putting a few drops of oil in hot water and then soaking a cloth in the mixture. Place compress on the bruises.

Alternatively, put a few drops in a carrier oil and massage into the bruise.

Allergies – Use a diffuser in your home or office during the day and during allergy season to help lesson symptoms. You can also spray on your feet and inhale directly during serious flares.

Irritability & Insomnia – Inhale or drink chamomile tea to help experience the calming effects of this essential oil.

Due to chamomile's anti-infectious, anti-inflammatory, anti-parasitic, calming and relaxing properties it's a very commonly used essential oil.

Eucalyptus

This essential oil is an analgesic, antibacterial, anti-inflammatory, insecticidal and expectant oil. Mostly used for respiratory issues due to the fragrant oil as well as the way the scent affects people psychologically.

Increase Circulation & Blood Flow – Put a drop in the massage oil and rub into skin to help increase circulation.

Improve Lung Function – Whether it's bronchitis, asthma or congestion you can improve the lung function by using an inhalation tent to breathe in the steam.

To Wakeup – Whether you have jet lag, trouble waking up in the morning or are just tired, adding some eucalyptus oil to your bath or shower can do wonders for your energy level.

There are many other uses for eucalyptus oil too, such as helping with kidney stones, reducing pain, and more. You'll definitely want to keep this around regularly.

Lemon

There are so many uses for lemon essential oils. You can use it for many purposes including antiseptic, cleansing and healing.

Concentration – Put some lemon oil into lotion so that you can rub it on your arms and neck, inhaling deeply. Then take a test, or do work. You'll find that your focus is better and your mind is sharper.

Alertness – If you feel as if you're dragging through the day and not really aware of what is happening around you, try inhaling some lemon oil using a diffuser in the room you're working in.

Positivity – Put some drops of lemon oil in candle wax, turn on some positive music and you'll feel a lot less negative almost immediately.

Nausea – If you're suffering from nausea due to morning sickness or as a side effect to medication try putting a few drops of lemon oil onto a cotton ball and sniff it each time you are afflicted.

Lemon is so common that you'll notice it's in so many things that you use from shampoo, to skin care, to cleaning products. That's because the smell is so clean and fresh and inoffensive.

These are likely some of the most commonly used essential oils. There are many others that you can use to get started with aromatherapy. Studying scents and how they can affect your health and quality of life can make a lot of difference in your life. You can use essential oils in so many ways to help improve and complement other methods of health care. Used wisely, you can accomplish so much more than you ever thought.

Resources

Below are suggested listings for a starter essential oil kit, diffuser and warming candle. Copy and paste the link of each item to view more information or to order.

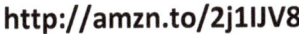

http://amzn.to/2j1IJV8

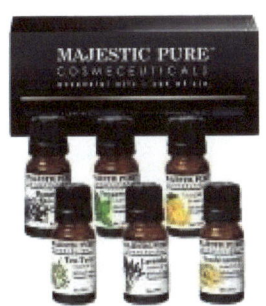

Essential Oils Set of Premium 6 from Majestic Pure, Therapeutic Grade Aromatherapy Oil Gift Set - 10 ml - Lavender, Frankincense, Peppermint, Lemon, Tea Tree & Rosemary Oils

Essential oils are used in range from aromatherapy, personal beauty care and natural treatments. Includes all components of famous thieves blend - Lavender, Frankincense, Peppermint, Lemon, Tea Tree and Rosemary Oils:
• Lavender – helps eliminate nervous tension, relieve pain, disinfect the scalp and skin, enhance blood circulation & alleviate respiratory problems
• Frankincense – helps relieve chronic stress & anxiety, reducing pain & inflammation, boosting immunity
• Peppermint - gives a cooling sensation, has a calming effect on the body which can relieve sore muscles
• Lemon – has stimulating, calming, carminative, anti-infection, astringent, detoxifying, antiseptic, disinfectant, sleep inducing, & antifungal properties
• Tea Tree – Helps with acnes, chickenpox, cold sores, athlete's foot, toenail fungus, jock itch, insect bites & sunburns
• Rosemary – helps promote hair growth, slows graying, alleviates dandruff and dry scalp

http://amzn.to/2j1BWee

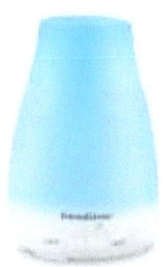

InnoGear Aromatherapy Essential Oil Diffuser Portable Ultrasonic Diffusers with Color LED Lights Changing and Waterless Auto Shut-off Function for Home Office Bedroom Room, 100 mL

This is perfect for small to medium sized rooms. Keeping your living space humid helps prevent colds/flu and congestion.

Hit the light button to transforms through 7 colors like a rainbow or stays on the color of your choice.

Features:
Three Settings toggled by the Mist button (Green/Red/Off):
* Green - intermittent mist (Mist 30 seconds and Pause 30 seconds)
* Red - continuous mist
* Off- You may use it as a color changing light without mist
Auto shut off when water runs out.
Keep essential oil 100% natural without burning or heating.

http://amzn.to/2j1L7Ln

Set of 2 Home Decorative Moon & Stars Black Ceramic Aromatherapy Burner / Essential Oil Warmer Candle Holder

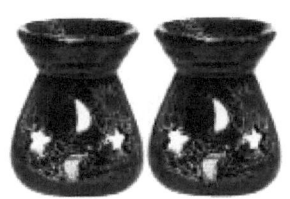

Bring style, warm candlelight and your favorite fragrance to any space with this set of 2 ceramic oil warmers. Just set a tea light candle inside each candle holder, light it, and add some of your chosen home fragrance oil to the small bowl on top. As the oil warms, the lovely fragrance and the soft candlelight will create warm, relaxing mood that will turn your home into a place for you to unwind and de-stress. The ceramic warmers have a glossy glaze and designed to look like marble giving these charming aroma diffuser a contemporary feel. The open work design of stars and moons beautifully glows with the warmth of candlelight.

Other Relevant Books by This Author

If you would like to read more relevant books about this topic, here is a list of the CreateSpace links, titles and descriptions from this author:

https://www.createspace.com/6750664

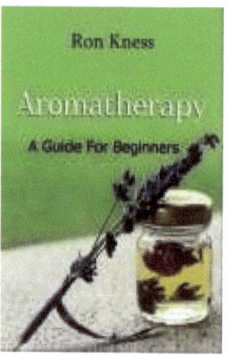

Aromatherapy – A Guide for Beginners

Are you looking for a natural alternative when it comes to your home and your life?

Have you looked at Aromatherapy products? If not, now is great time to stop and take a closer look.

If you have not considered using aromatherapy in your life, you are not alone. Hundreds of others are looking at how they too can improve not just their homes, but their health and that of their family – including their pets – by using aromatherapy and essential oils.

No doubt your grandmothers used oils in many different ways. To help freshen their air in their homes, for putting into the bath tub, or under their pillows to help induce sleep.

If this worked for them, why won't it work for you today? Not sure what aromatherapy is, and how it can help you? Well, today you are in the right place at the right time!

Inside you will discover answers to your most pressing questions on this popular topic
- Why is quality so important with essential oils?
- What is aromatherapy?
- Can I use aromatherapy and essential oils on my pets?
- What's the best way to store essential oils?
- How long do essential oils last?
- Are essential oils safe to take internally?
And more...

Aromatherapy - A Guide for Beginners will help you understand what essential oils are, and how you can use them safely.

It's important to understand what oils to choose, and to know what oils are best suited for specific purposes.
- Lavender is perfect as a soothing oil and to freshen the air in your home.
- Peppermint will help relax you and is great when used as a tea.
- Ginger helps your circulation and is great for massaging joints and helping those dealing with arthritis.
- Sandalwood helps with skin issues, bronchitis, stress & stretch marks.

Aromatherapy and the use of essential oils is on the increase. People around the world are searching for natural alternatives that are better suited for their health, their wallet and the environment.

https://www.createspace.com/5714434

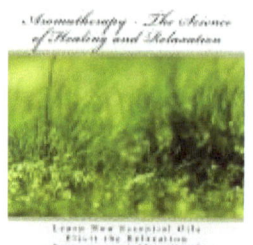

Aromatherapy – The Science of Healing and Relaxation

In this book, we reveal the natural holistic methods issues and to relive stress through relaxation.

In particular we talk about:
• Aromatherapy - what it is and how it works
• Essential Oils – how the effects of certain aromas differs from others
• Recipes – how to make your own essential oil combinations

Aromatherapy

The results of The American Psychological Association's 2010 Stress in America survey showed that nearly 75% of Americans who responded to the survey believe their stress levels to be so high that they feel unhealthy. Stress and anxiety reflect the reaction of the body and the mind when over stimulated.

Stress tends to reflect the physical responses of the body when coping with daily pressures, physical labor, a high-paced work environment, toxic relationships, and financial and emotional responsibilities, which exceed a person's ability to cope or manage. However, your sense of smell can help relieve stress by smelling certain aromas.

Essential Oils

When selecting oils to combat anxiety and stress, choose oils with relaxing, calming, and uplifting properties. The oils should soothe while shifting the awareness in a way that grounds and replenishes the constitution of the person being treated. The scents that work best for anxiety and stress relief tend to have light and bright floral, citrus, or woodsy scents.

The essential oils recommended for relaxation and mood adjustment may be blended with those recommended for managing stress and anxiety. Many of them are complementary scents with complementary therapeutic qualities.

Recipes

There are many ways to enjoy the benefits of essential oils. When selecting a method of application, the issue being treated must be considered along with the desired results.

For example:
==> Creams, ointments, and gels work best for treating injuries like bruises and cuts.
==> A massage oil works well for treating muscle aches and pains.
==> If the primary purpose of the treatment is to shift a person's mood in some way, incense or a diffuser may be the best option.

While you can buy certain combinations of oils, we include in our book several recipes and show you how you can make a unique essential oil tailored just to you.

"Aromatherapy – The Science of Healing and Relaxation" is a

must-have book for those that are overstressed and starting to exhibit the effects of stress either through the development of physical or mental responses, or both. What you smell can make you feel better!

About the Author

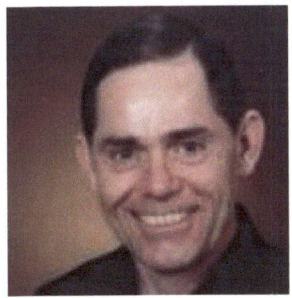

I grew up in Central Minnesota, where my parents owned and operated a fishing resort. Once out of high school I tried a couple of semesters of college, only to quit halfway through the Spring term; I decided at that time that college wasn't for me.

Then I decided to follow my father's previous occupation as an auto mechanic. I graduated from a two-year of vocational training course and worked as a mechanic for five years. While in vocational training, I decided to join the National Guard where I eventually ended up working full-time for 32 years.

So how does all of this relate to writing? In one of my leadership schools, the instructor, who was an English teacher at a juvenile detention center, presented writing to me in a whole new way - a way that started to develop my interest in working with words.

I eventually went back to college on the GI Bill while I was working and earned my Bachelor's degree in Business Administration. Taking a class or two per semester at night and on weekends took me seven years to complete my degree.

Fast forward about 40 years and I now have published over 100 books on Amazon for Kindle, CreateSpace and other publishing platforms.

Besides my own writing, I also ghostwrite ebooks, books, reports, articles, blogs and do Kindle conversions for clients on a variety of topics.

Today my wife and I are retired from our careers and live in Gold Canyon, AZ. I now write as a retirement business where you'll find me happily sitting in my office typing away on my laptop as I work on my next book or ghostwriting project . . . that is if we are not traveling on a cruise ship - our new-found mode of travel.

www.ingramcontent.com/pod-product-compliance
Lightning Source LLC
Chambersburg PA
CBHW050822290526
45792CB00001B/219